Published
Author and the publisher www.ebooksolutions.org.

All Rights Reserved. No part of this publication may be reproduced in any form or by any means, including scanning, photocopying, or otherwise without prior written permission of the copyright holder.

Disclaimer and Terms of Use: The Author and Publisher have strived to be as accurate and complete as possible in the creation of this book, notwithstanding the fact that he does not warrant or represent at any time that the contents within are accurate due to the rapidly changing nature of the internet. While all attempts have been made to verify information provided in the publication, the Author and Publisher assumes no responsibility for errors, omissions, or contrary interpretation of the subject matter herein. Any perceived slights of specific persons, peoples, or organizations are unintentional. In practical advice books, like anything else in life, there are not guarantees of income made. This book is not intended for use as a source of legal, business, accounting or financial advice. All readers are advised to seek services of competent professionals in legal, business, accounting, and finance fields.

This book is designed to give correct and helpful information. While all attempts have been made to verify the information provided in this publication, neither the Author nor the Publisher assumes any responsibility for errors, omissions, or contrary interpretation of the subject matter herein. The Author and the Publisher are not doctors and make no attempt to diagnose, cure or prevent any disease. The contents of this book should not be treated as a substitute for the medical advice of your own doctor or any other health care professional. This publication is intended as an information product only. The purchaser or reader of this publication assumes all responsibility for the use of these materials, and information. The Author and Publisher assume no responsibility or liability whatsoever on behalf of the purchaser or reader of these materials.

Contents

Introduction..5
- Acid and Alkaline......................................10
- Measuring pH...15
- PARASITES, pH balance, and how this impacts you!..20
- PREMATURE AGING, ph balance, and how this impacts you!..24
- CANCER, ph balance, and how this affects you!..28
- DIABETES, pH balance, and how this affects you!..32
- EXCESSIVE DAIRY, pH balance, and how this affects you!..36
- SUGAR, pH balance, and how this affects you!..40
- STRESS, pH balance, and how this affects you!..45
- Getting more Alkaline into your diet............48
- Cooking tips for your pH balanced diet.........52
- Green Drinks for your pH balanced diet........56
- Water Ionizers and your pH balanced diet....60
- Shopping tips for your pH balanced diet.......64
- Common Mistakes people make with a pH balanced diet..68

Conclusion..72

Introduction

I want you to be happy and healthy! You may be asking yourself, "What does a book about balancing my body's pH have to do with being happy and healthy?" If you are asking yourself that question, it will be answered shortly! Back to your happiness and health J.

To be sure we are all looking at things from the same point of view, I want to define two important terms: happy and healthy. www.merriam-webster.com defines happy as "enjoying or characterized by well-being and contentment". Merriam-Webster defines health as "the condition of being sound in body, mind, or spirit; especially: freedom from physical disease or pain." By looking at these two definitions, it is pretty safe to infer that someone who is happy is more likely to do the things to take care of themselves and be healthy than someone who is unhappy. Haven't we all seen someone who has had something happen in their life, a bad breakup for example, and that person does not want to do anything? They stay home, eat a lot of junk food, don't care about their appearance, etc. The general care one typically has for his/her own well-being is reduced during unhappy times.

The definition of health-specifically the part that says "the condition of being sound in body, mind, or spirit-" denotes a link to happiness!

If we are overweight and the clothes we once wore no longer fit, this probably won't make us happy. Additionally, the extra weight has potential health consequences that should be put in check.

If we are stuck at home, under the weather because of the flu or a cold, there is a good chance that we are not happy in that situation. Clearly, health and happiness go hand-in-hand.

In two reports created by JWT Intelligence titled "JWT:10 Trends for 2013" and "Health & Happiness: Hand in Hand," they examine the relationship between these two states of being. As I touched on a few sentences ago, the notion of health is being viewed holistically, to encompass mind and body. The idea of health and happiness being related is not a new concept; there is more statistical evidence that supports this notion. For example, in their "Health & Happiness: Hand in Hand" report, they cite research that states that optimistic people are up to 50% LESS LIKELY to suffer a heart attack or stroke. The research also shows that negative mental states, such as anxiety or anger, can negatively affect cardiac health. WOW!

This report even lists foods we eat that contribute to our mental health. For example, the Mental Health Foundation has a report that links the debilitating condition of depression with junk foods and diets lacking general nutritional elements. In the book titled The Happiness Diet, the author's research shows that the modern US diet is not only unhealthy; It also has attributes that can lead towards a depressed and anxious lifestyle. In keeping with one of the themes in this book, it can also be said that this diet causes the body to slide in the direction of acidity. The consequences of an acidic diet will be explored later in the book.

An article published in the Huffington Post supports the research presented above. In a survey that looked at 18 countries and ranked the most depressed to least, the US was the second most depressed country.

China was the least depressed. In contrast to the US diet, a Chinese diet tends to lean more towards neutral and alkalinity, which can result in more benefits to a person's overall health and happiness.

Going back to the question you may have been asking yourself earlier, which is "What does a book about balancing my body's pH have to do with being happy and healthy?" In my personal opinion (and we all have one!), I believe that the steps and processes involved in balancing your body's pH will not only make your insides healthy; It will introduce you to a diet that WILL provide your body with nutritional elements that will boost your happiness! I believe this approach will provide an optimal "one-two punch" to the happiness and health I have been talking about.

The book **pH Balance** has information inside it that, if followed, will make you remarkably healthier, which, in turn, will contribute to your overall happiness! This book focuses a lot on the food that you eat and impacts that it can have in your life. The age old adage "You are what you eat" is really examined in **pH Balance.** What I hope you learn in this book is that many of the "bad" foods that we eat are doing more to our body than adding a few pounds and causing cholesterol levels to rise and that some of the foods that we eat-which are typically deemed as a "good" food-can actually be doing more harm than good!

As a final note, the concepts discussed in **pH Balance** are not meant to provide you with a particular dieting fad or trend. There are already a lot of good diet plans available. I will say however, that if you follow the advice provided in this book, you will begin taking steps towards an eating lifestyle that will complement and enhance other diet programs.

Thank you once again for taking the time to read this book. I hope you are able to gain something valuable. When you finish the book, please leave a review and provide your feedback. I cannot wait to see it. Enjoy your read!

Acid and Alkaline

The main reason for you to start a diet which focuses on pH balance is to preserve a balance of pH in the foods you consume. Since the human body is a bit alkaline, then in the end it is better for your health and wellness that you eat a diet made up of alkalizing meals. Anytime you eat a lot of acidic meals, your system gets out of balance, thereby creating a lot of complications such as weight increase, insufficient focus and fatigue, in addition to a low immunity which leads to a lot of other crucial conditions.

A diet focusing on pH balance depends on lists of acidic meals (to be avoided) as well as alkalizing meals (to be emphasized). The alkalizing meals are better for your health and wellness and in addition help balance your body's pH. Although acid, alkaline and pH are familiar terms, many people do not get exactly what they mean and how they relate to health, nutrition and wellness.

"Basic" as a word comes from "basis", a Classical word which refers to base. "Basic" refers to acidity and alkalinity properties. These conditions start from the root foundation of our body cells which the meals we consume are composed of. Therefore, an external influence makes no difference to the acidity or alkalinity of a food. Rather, foods are acid or alkaline at their foundation.

Acid and alkaline are naturally opposite chemical substances. When a base interacts with an acid, a battle occurs between them leading to the formation of sodium.

It's a simple interaction in the lab of a chemist but in our bodies, it becomes far more complex as result of the scope at which acids and bases contact.

Science, however, can generalize the outcomes of acids and alkaline in the digestive systems of human beings. Acidic foods form acids in the body. They make our blood, our saliva and our lymph much more acidic, leading to a reduced pH value in our body. Alkaline meals on the other hand make them more alkaline thereby leading to a higher pH value.

For the sake of reference, the range considered "normal" for the pH of saliva is between 7.3 and 7.4. A lot of people, however, are very acidic, having a pH much lower. Their bodies are therefore burned out, weary and in dare need of good balance. Under the effect of acidic foods your muscles wear down rapidly causing your body to basically slow down as a result of being unable to make the very same physical results as they did before.

When we consume acidic foods, free radical oxidation occurs, leading to quicker aging. Minerals and supplements are not absorbed as normally as they would be. Those friendly germs in the small intestine become dead because of this, leading to imbalance in the digestive system. What causes further damage to the small intestine operation is the fact that a lot of acidity prevents the ability of the abdominal wall surfaces to absorb good nutrients. This leads to cells becoming strained because of the developed toxins in addition to an inability to expel them. A lot of functions in the body can no longer run at their optimum capacity.

On the contrary, alkaline foods have a large variety of advantages for you in terms of health and wellness. Consumption of alkaline foods increases our muscle output. They also have antioxidant effects in our body. They accelerate our assimilation down to the cellular level and make the cells operate in the right manner. Using alkaline foods causes a reduction of parasites and overgrowth of yeast. Alkaline foods encourages better and more relaxed rest, gives us younger looking skin and relieve us of cold symptoms, flu and headaches. Alkaline foods advance our physical energy abundantly.

Perhaps the most crucial differences between alkaline and acidic foods are the way they relate to cancer. Cancerous tissues are widely acidic and healthy ones alkaline. When oxygen is introduced to an acidic solution, it combines with hydrogen ions in the acid to form water easily. While oxygen helps in reducing the effects of the acid, the acid hinders oxygen from getting to tissues where it is required. When air enters an alkaline solution, the two hydroxyl ions combine with the solution, creating one molecule of water and one atom of air. The lone oxygen atom is released to the next cell and delivers the benefits of air to all body tissue. At a pH value slightly above 7.4, cancer cells get inactive. Researches reveal that when pH reaches 8.5, cancer cells die while healthy and balanced cells thrive.

Alkalizing your diet provides a lot of benefits, as well as helping you to avoid cancer. A list of alkaline food is a form of selections that will surely provide benefits to your health when your body starts using them.

Measuring pH

Were you aware that your blood has a pH level? pH is the measure of exactly how acidic or alkaline a substance is. The scale for the measurement of pH level runs from 1 to 14, 1 being associated with "very acidic", 7 being "neutral" and 14 meaning "incredibly alkaline". In actual fact, your circulatory system goes to the extent of preserving its pH level between 7.30 and 7.40 which is somewhat alkaline. Why is this crucial? One of the many reasons why your body maintains this balance starts with your energy level. By maintaining a diet focusing on pH balance, you are assisting your body to balance and your energy to increase.

Have you ever filled a lower quality fuel in your vehicle tank after running it previously on premium fuel? You most likely noticed a difference in the vehicle acceleration, handling, and its general performance. This has a direct connection with the quality of fuel you filled in the tank. Your body is like a finely tuned machine. Machines need their parts to be kept running by fuel. The best fuel for your body is a custom mixture which is even more alkaline than acid. But what difference exactly does this make?

It is in the bloodstream that it all starts. Look at the bloodstream as a superhighway having stops all over your body. Red blood cells are the moving traffic which rides along the bloodstream in a haste to get to work. Each of these red blood cells has a negative charge on it, and this prevents them from getting into fender benders and sudden crashes in the circulatory system.

When these negative charges get stripped from the red blood cells, they cluster together and can easily cause "traffic jam" and bottlenecks in the bloodstream. Put another way, the traffic movement in the bloodstream isn't really efficient and this causes things to slowdown. If you've ever experienced getting stuck in freeway traffic then you understand just how irritating it is.

This impact on the body triggers a domino effect, which ultimately depletes your energy, making you tired and sluggish. Acid is the culprit in the bloodstream traffic jam! When acid is added to your circulatory system it bites off the negative charge surrounding each red blood cell and creates different kinds of problems. But how exactly can you prevent this? The simple and straightforward solution starts with what you put into your stomach. It is what we eat that develops red blood cells. When your stomach absorbs the food, it leaves behind natural acidic waste and your body expels this waste through your urine and sweat. Nevertheless, a point comes when the waste accumulation is too much to get rid of.

Then what does your body do with all of the acidic waste it cannot remove? The answer is a little shocking: it stores it in your body! Since the cells in your body are naturally alkaline, the addition of this acid waste starts to attack and ruin them. A lot of energy is expelled in the process of trying to keep the waste from doing further harm to your body. However, this battle goes on for a long time. In the end, the acid buildup is so tremendous that the cells decline, creating energy depletion and leaving the body exposed to illness.

How exactly can you prevent this slow death? A Higher energy level helps to prevent unfortunate illnesses and ensures solid cellular regeneration. Altering your diet is a great step in changing this breakdown of your body and simultaneously enhancing your energy level. The choice of food you take will drastically reveal exactly how much of acidic waste are stored in your body. The more alkaline the food you choose, the less the quantity of acidic waste that will be stored in your body, tipping the balance in the favor of sound health for yourself.

As the old adage says, you are what you eat and this is absolutely true. Controlling the amount of alkaline food you put in your body will help give your body a chance to fight. By limiting your intake of acidic foods and raising your intake of alkaline food, you are increasing your stamina easily, getting more endurance and overall functioning of your body appliance.

One of the quickest ways to get an idea of your pH is to use something called pH strips. They are small strips of litmus paper that allow someone to get a quick a idea of where their pH level is on the overall pH scale. The results typically come back in a matter of seconds and from there, one can begin making the proper adjustments (if necessary) based off of the advice given in this book.

Here is a list of various pH strips you can browse through (pH strips). After finding the pH strips you want, make sure you take your measurement and begin making the right decisions to improve your quality of life today!

PARASITES, pH balance, and how this impacts you!

A diet focusing on pH balance restores balance to your body. By consuming mainly alkaline foods, your body will receive nutrition that conforms to the alkaline state of your body cells. Consuming too much acidic foods can easily cause a host of issues. In addition to other advantages, following a diet focusing on pH balance can lower your body's tendency to keep harmful parasites in your system which can destroy your health.

Is there any connection between pH and parasites? At the intracellular level, the human body has a usual pH of about 7.4 which is alkaline somewhat. Parasites, which consists of are harmful germs, tiny worms, amoebas, viruses, and protozoa cannot easily survive in any medium with a pH between 7.3 and 7.4.

In America, there's a diet which creates high levels of acid at the intracellular level. It is called acidosis, and is a main hidden source to many conditions. In addition, it gives room for parasites to spread widely through your body. If you would like to be healthy, you must bring balance back to your body by taking an alkalizing diet.

With time, everything you consume either leaves your bodies in an acidic state or an alkaline state. Starches and refined sugars, both of which are an important mainstay of the Western diet, are among the perpetrators of the acidification procedure. Sources of natural sugar contain vitamins and minerals in them. Though fruits initially contained acids, they have the required minerals which help the cells to turn their acids into alkaline by-products.

Refined (processed) sugars do not, and when they are consumed, they introduce acid into the body. Substantial consumption of sugars and starches make the body to become acidic.

At the intracellular level, acidic pH becomes a safe haven for parasites and really creates a mutation of friendly intestinal flora, thereby causing a condition called candidiasis. Candida is the name of a natural yeast living in the intestine and is balanced by friendly bacteria living with it.

However, overuse of sugar and the introduction of antibiotics will certainly make these friendly micro-organisms less common. Candida will undergo mutation and grow until it is out of control. Some of the signs of Candida fungus are unmanageable sugar cravings, dry skin, stubborn yeast infections, fatigue, regular sinus infections and acne. When yeast flourishes, even parasites can because there are no friendly micro-organisms to keep them in control. Worms that would normally pass through the body have now discovered a favorable environment and take control of the intestine.

Parasites can destroy and damage cells at a speed much faster than that with which they can be regenerated. In addition, they create harmful substances which are by-product of their food digestions. These deadly substances can produce allergic reactions and can easily cause you to develop brand-new allergic reactions to food. Parasites can even invade and worsen your body tissues, and infect the intestinal coating and the skin. The parasites create a challenging environment for the tissues to operate correctly.

With time, organs can become blocked, leading to pressure development in your body organs and all body operations. Immune system depression sets in and the presence of parasites can easily hinder the ability of your body to have natural recovery reactions. Ultimately, presence of too many parasites can easily lead your body into the problem of inappropriate nutrient absorption.

The best solution is to follow a diet which focuses on pH balance. This will help you to easily repair your body's balance. Because of the fact that parasites cannot survive in any environment having a pH between 7.3 and 7.4, taking alkaline diet will help you eliminate them from your system. Following this diet will provide you the ability to invert the acidification process and turn your body to an inhabitable environment for parasites.

PREMATURE AGING, ph balance, and how this impacts you!

A lot of people think immediately of fat burning when they hear the word "diet". The focus we have on thinness in our culture makes us to relate this word with shedding some weight. On the contrary, we are defining a diet as any sort of foods or drinks we put into our body. Your overall wellness is affected greatly by the diet you eat. A diet which focuses on pH balance is not just a diet that burns fat. If your diet is not pH balanced, it can cause you many problems. One of which is the physical effects of aging on your body.

Precisely what has aging got to do with pH and an acid or alkaline food? A few professionals argue that the reason we experience physical aging has to do completely with the quantity of acidic foods that we put into our body. The point is that we grow older because we do not efficiently eject those wastes and contaminants collected through our bodies.

Nutrients are burned within our cells to release energy, maintain our body temperatures and make our bodies function correctly. No matter what sort of food we consume, whether acid or alkaline, veggie or meat, healthy or unhealthy food, they contain exactly the same elements namely carbon, hydrogen, nitrogen and air.

So as to work correctly, the cells have to use these nutrients. They "oxidize" or break the nutrients down to natural acids namely carbonic acids, lactic acids, uric acids and fatty acids. These acids are removed by the cells in their waste form through our sweat and urine. When the body operates correctly and in a well-balanced manner, there are no problems with these waste acids. They can be conveniently and easily eliminated by the body making you to easily maintain a typical pH of 7.4 or close.

Unfortunately, the modern way in which we live has really affected the capacity of our bodies to properly get rid of the acids from them. Insufficient rest, shortage of workouts, excessive labor, getting worried, smoking of cigarettes, pollution of air and taking high acidic diets containing too much of meat and dairy products, all hinder our bodies from properly removing these acids. This way of life leads to the production of excessive acids which the body therefore struggles to get rid of this excess.

The situation is even worsened by the practices of the modern-day farming and food development which make foods more acidic than they should normally be. Some inorganic acid minerals such as phosphor, chlorine, and sulfur leak into meats. They also find their way into our grains and root crops via the ground soil. The quality of air and farming practices are more reasons of this upsurge in inorganic acid minerals. We now consume far more inorganic acid minerals than ever before. What all this does is to make our bodies unable to free themselves of acid.

Our over-acidified lives are creating premature aging and an ideal solution is to take diets which focus on pH balance. We age because we accumulate acidic elements in our body. Cells which are balanced and healthy naturally have a little bit of alkaline pH degree, and for the fact that acid and alkaline are opposite chemicals, high levels of acid destroy living cells.

To stop the effects of rapid aging and reverse the effects of acidic damage on our cells, we must start alkalizing our diets in accordance with diets which focus on pH balance. We need to assist our bodies to develop a good system which will help it purge itself of acid wastes. We must facilitate pulling old wastes away from your body.

The first step to take is we should drink a lot of water, particularly acid -free alkaline water. Only 4 glasses of alkaline water are far more effective than 8 glasses of ordinary water. We can use water ionizers to help us develop alkaline water in the convenience of our homes. The purpose of this water is to help us flush out our system and remove the accumulation of acidity inside.

A diet which focuses on pH balance promotes the consumption of a greater portion of alkaline foods in our diet. The alkalizing foods will definitely help in the restoration of balance to our body and remove the rest of the accumulated acid waste. The outcomes of this are that we will have younger appearance, become more energetic and have a relief from some symptoms of aging such as arthritis.

CANCER, ph balance, and how this affects you!

A most important point of a diet which focuses on pH balance is that the principles of the diet can be applied to prevent and turn around cancer. Although these statements are debatable in the sphere of fitness and wellness, there are individuals whose cancer and general level of wellness have been reversed because they consume diets which are focused on pH balance. This book is not meant to replace any sound medical advice. **DISCLAIMER! As always, please consult with a medical doctor regarding your medical needs. DISCLAIMER!**

Dr. Robert Young, the person who made the pH miracle diet, says cancer is not really a condition or illness as we generally think but an outcome of the metabolic acids which are developed in the blood then deposited in the tissues. Cancer, Dr. Young says, is actually an acidic liquid which spills into living cells, tissues and body organs and not a mutation of the cells.

Every condition originates from a source. Cancer has clear and straight sources, and as demonstrated by of a diet focusing on pH balance, the cause for cancer is found in over acidity. Illnesses such as cancer are caused by systemic acidosis, which results in very low pH (less than 7.4). Any pH value below 7.0 is considered acidic, and the lower the value of the pH, the greater the acidity level or degree in the body.

On the cellular scale, your cells absorb the food you consume and produce metabolic acids. Those acids are in general ejected by your body through your sweat or urine. When you take a large amount of acidic foods and live a very acidic lifestyle your body knows not what to do with the remaining acid waste. When you take very acidic foods normally, there is inadequate energy which your body can use to get rid the excess acids. These acids therefore collect in your body, and disrupt cellular activities.

Initially, metabolic acids are first stored in the blood but later transferred to and stored in the tissues. While they are in the tissue, metabolic acids cause illness, sickness and cancerous tissues. Cancer is the acidic product of metabolism that collects in the body, impacting the cells around it and, more or less like a rotten apple in a barrel, consequently spreads from one cell to another causing disease. Cancer is not born by mutated cells. The cells themselves do not change their form however there is restriction of their function as a result of the existence of excess metabolic acid. There is nothing like "cancer cells". They are typical cells which have become extremely acidic.

Among the strangest part of the relationship between pH and cancer is that tumors are really attempting to help the body. They form in places where the metabolic acid is widespread and effect cellular feature. Tumors are attempts in your body for preventing the spread out of the acidic cells to other parts of your body. In fact the tumor is a signal telling you where your body collects excess metabolic acid. Some people are genetically adapted to collect metabolic acid in particular spots in the body. This is why there is history of a certain type of cancer in some families, for example, breast cancer.

The tumors are not the complication on their own. They only indicate precisely what is failing in a given part of the body. When cancer metastasizes, it is an indication that the acidic condition is proceeding to affect some other cells, making them too acidic.

Cancer is not something that we get unanticipated. Formation of cancer in our body is a sign of the decisions we have taken about what we consume and exactly how we live our lives. An alkaline manner of life focusing on an alkaline diet and other soothing habits are surely less likely to cause cancer. An acidic manner of life and diet will certainly contain the pains of the development of metabolic acid which, in extreme cases, can lead to cancer.

That is great news because it implies that cancer can be prevented and treated. A cancer patient can easily start taking steps which will help him or her to change the effects of cancer and prevent its spread. He or she should consume an alkaline centered diet which is more aggressive than that of someone who is only attempting to acquire better total wellness. However, by adopting the principles of a diet which is focused on pH balance, they can eventually succeed in their struggle to reduce, control and remove cancer completely from their bodies.

DIABETES, pH balance, and how this affects you!

The third leading source of fatalities in the US is diabetic issues. What is more shocking is the fact that, diabetes is a top cause of fatality among young children. Considering the increasing number of people gaining too much weight in this country, it has produced increasing number of cases of type II diabetes (also called adult onset diabetes). Presently, one person in every 12 people is affected with the illness. This means over 16 million people are suffering from this condition out of which 6 million are left undiagnosed and not aware of their sensitive insulin status.

Issues of Type II diabetic are caused by obesity, high tension, poor nutrition, increased aging, and general physical inactivity. All of these conditions are attributed to only one source: high levels of acidity! Hyper-acid lifestyles and food selections have negative impacts on our wellness, as shown by the rapid increase in the rate of diabetes in the country.

Diabetic is a very old ailment because it was discovered hundreds of years ago, yet it is only in the modern day that it has turned to an epidemic. What causes part of this complication is that the nature of diabetic issues has remained a mystery, even to civilized people. Many people do not understand precisely what insulin does in our body and how exactly the metabolic rate of insulin affects our health. Even modern medical science misinterprets the real nature of the disorder.

For instance, many medical practitioners believe that the reason for diabetes is excessive weight. On the other hand, weight problems are a result of increased consumption of simple sugars and complicated carbohydrates. The alarming rate of consumption of these products, which are manufactured from acidifying foods like sugar and processed wheat, introduces high level of acidity to the body. Hence, the body tries to control the increased amount of waste acids by using fat to neutralize the acids. To safeguard the cells in the body, the fat is then stored.

There are other people who believe that insulin is required for the regulation of blood sugar levels in the body. The phrase "insulin dependent" was coined in the '50s to give the impression that muscle and fat require insulin to break down sugar, that is, the sugars produced by taking sweet and high carbohydrate and foods. Nevertheless, modern researches reveal that many different things in our body transport glucose. Cells demand for glucose for their respiration. The body ensures that the cells receive the glucose, regardless of how much insulin is present in it.

Insulin resistance, which leads to type II diabetes, is encouraged by a very acidic lifestyle and choices of acidic foods. It takes place in our livers, muscles and fat cells. Having too much caffeine, sugar, chocolate and carbohydrates stimulate the mentioned organs and tissues. This stimulation causes the cells to start releasing their glucose, leading to the elevated blood sugar levels observed during blood glucose testing. The body cells become disorganized and their terrible acidic state can trigger a lot of issues with time, leading to premature aging, hypertension, difficulty in releasing glycogen from the liver, and inhibition of fat burning.

Excessive stimulation of the bodily tissues through consumption of acidic foods can cause a lot of damage, and type II diabetic issues are only an indication of an acidic lifestyle. In order to restore balance back to the body, you should adopt a diet containing alkalizing green vegetables, green beverages and excellent fats. Plant proteins obtained from grains and legumes also help to return the body's former equilibrium. A diet focusing on pH balance contains a balanced strategy for eating with your body and not against it. The application of the ideas of this type of diet will make the control and prevention of diabetic issues an easy matter of alkalized consumption and living.

EXCESSIVE DAIRY, pH balance, and how this affects you!

Diets focusing on pH balance attempt check many conditions in our body, including obesity, omitting acidifying foods and conducts. Among the most surprising additions on the list, at least to a Westerner, is milk. Although dairy products may be a mainstay of the Western diet, they are not a part of global populations' diets. So what precisely does the rest of the world know that we don't? From a pH point of view, dairy is not needed for wellness but actually does harm to the body.

Many people believe that milk and dairy products are essential for bone density and our overall wellness. However, dairy products have ample quantities of protein and fat, both of which are nothing but acid forming elements. Cow's milk and its derivatives form acid but cheeses and milk obtained from goat and sheep have less fat and protein and form less acid. The only exception is clarified butter which is alkalizing because of the short chain fats in it.

Around 2003, the Harvard School of Public Health gave an alternative pyramid to the FDA suggestions because of imbalances seen by members in the former pyramid. Though it did not talk about acid and alkaline foods in particular, the pyramid displays a tendency to alkaline foods. A most important difference between the FDA pyramid and that of Harvard is the addition of a dairy serving or calcium supplement once daily. The FDA suggests two to three servings every day, in addition to dietary supplements.

Calcium is needed by the body but not at the levels found in the 2 to 3 servings which were encouraged by the FDA. Calcium is needed for normal development of bone and its maintenance yet the average adult can easily obtain sufficient calcium from supplements. The quantity of calcium in 2 to 3 daily servings of dairy can in actual fact be harmful to wellness. Consumption of too much calcium may raise your risk for some cancers and no links have been found between large quantities of calcium and osteoporosis prevention.

In addition, dairy is never a pure food. The dairy sector has really endeavored to increase cow's milk image by saying it is crucial and beneficial. Remember however, that 50 years ago the typical cow produced 2,000 pounds of milk yearly while the modern cows normally produce 50,000 pounds a year. Prescription antibiotics, drugs, focused breeding, forced feeding and hormones, all contribute to increasing milk processing so that dairy farmers can produce in large quantities. All of the above mentioned additives are part of the milk that everybody drinks daily.

A growing number of Americans, among whom are those following a diet focusing on pH balance, are removing dairy from their diet and getting amazing outcomes. The result of recent studies shows that milk is linked to anemia, intestinal irritation, intestinal colic and allergic reactions in very young and grown up children. In children, the primary complications found were allergy, asthma, colic, ear and tonsil infections and youth diabetes. The studies revealed that people had arthritis, heart disease, sensitivity and sinusitis because they consumed conventionally produced milk.

If you make a quick simple search for the dangers of dairy, you will be better educated about this so called "safe" food. If you check out the outcome of the research you will find out that it is the acidic nature of milk and other dairy items that tells us why milk is reduced and in some cases completely removed in diets focusing on pH balance.

SUGAR, pH balance, and how this affects you!

A diet focusing on pH balance emphasizes a well balanced approach to eating. As already discussed in previous chapters, we can easily achieve ideal wellness by limiting the consumption of acidic meals and increasing the consumption of alkaline meals. Sugar is one of the main factors in our battle against acidic pH levels. Sugar is an epidemic in our today's world. The average American consumes 2 to 3 pounds of sugar every week, implying that over 135 pounds of sugar is consumed by individual per year. This upsetting number is caused by the wide usage of sugar as an additive. Sugar is in everything we consume, concealed in various foods. Dextrose, Sucrose and high fructose corn syrups are active components of all processed meals and flavors. These highly refined substances deposit a bitter taste in the mouths of people who are starting a diet focusing on pH balance because of their global acceptance as a "necessary evil'.

Because of the radical impact of sugar on insulin levels, the body has no "weapon" to fight against the damage. As our insulin levels drop so does the release of growth hormone. These growth hormones weaken the immune system leaving the body exposed to a host of illness conditions and maladies. Insulin also blocks the capacity of the body to fight off weight gain and increased triglyceride levels. In simpler language, the greater the quantity of simple sugars in our meals, the more likely it will increase fat storage in our body. These fat cells invite acidic waste which in turn weakens the framework of red blood cells in the bloodstream.

Moreover, sugar fights with vitamin C for control of the cellular development in the body. Looking from a structural point of view, Vitamin C and Simple Sugar are very similar. As sugar levels increase in the body, they compete with one another when they enter the cells. A higher concentration of sugar in the circulatory system will certainly allow more sugar to get into thirsty cells, leaving little or no space for Vitamin C. Without the defensive results of Vitamin C on cellular frameworks they cannot resist the attacks of infections and bacteria. A reduction in the number of white blood cell counts produces a suppressed immune system that is too weak to defend the body.

Sugar contains no vitamins and minerals and after its absorption needs the help of vital micro-nutrients to metabolize into the system. A deficit occurs in the system when these micro-nutrients are not replaced. This deficiency makes it difficult for fat cells and cholesterol to be metabolized, resulting in obesity and hypertension (or high blood pressure). The ability of sugar to increase insulin levels artificially will in the end leave the pancreas dysfunctional thereby making the body dependent on sugar. This is usually referred to as diabetic issues. Simple sugars have in addition caused gallstones, allergies, mood ailments, and cardiovascular disease. With all of these and more adverse results that are clinically connected to sugars, it is still surprising that sugar is also one of the most acidic things that are so easy to feed our body.

Cancer is the most risky outcome of over-dependence on sugar. Cancerous cells thrive on lactic acid. This lactic acid which is produced by fermenting glucose is transported into the liver. A more acidic PH is the result of this build up of lactic acid in the malignant cells, the highly acidic nature of cancerous cysts being a testament to this. The relationship between sugars and unwanted acidic levels in the bloodstream is clearly explained by the connection of glucose (sugar) and cancerous cells. Simple sugars are poisonous to the body and will in the end decrease the quality of cellular development and suppress the immune system until it fails to function.

By maintaining a balancing in the diet with an 80 per cent alkaline and 20 percent acid induction of meals, supplements, and refreshments you can reduce the danger of diseases in your body. If you can replace simple sugars with more complicated or alkaline-based sugars like Stevia, you will find it easy to decrease your reliance on easy sugars and prevent bad health. Study active ingredient labels and be familiar with the many names that simple sugars lurk behind. Enlighten yourself on just how your body metabolizes simple sugars and also how carbohydrates can be broken down to simple sugars in your circulatory system. By equipping yourself with all those details you can easily improve your health.

STRESS, pH balance, and how this affects you!

A diet that focusing on pH balance is an excellent way of considering exactly how you eat your food. You can negotiate a balance by monitoring each of your foods, beverages, supplements, and additives by their acidic or alkaline signature. As stated in earlier chapters, our bodies work in accordance with the pH scale, working on a variety of 1 to 14. On this scale, a rank of 1 represents a high degree of acid while a rank of 14 indicates that the presence of a high concentration of alkaline. A ranking of 7 on the pH scale represents a neutral pH. The human blood survives at the pH degree of 7.35, which is slightly alkaline. A diet focusing on pH balance keeps the meals you take into your body within this pH range. The method of implementation is very simple: if you synchronize meals around a comprehensive list of meals and supplements you can easily establish an effective technique for reducing acidity in your body.

Alkaline intake will definitely prevent stored acidity from being metabolized and will neutralize it at the source. Since balance is the standard for a workable health plan, consistent tracking of the body's pH levels is important. Using saliva pH examination strips having a base range of 4.5 to 8.5 will allow you to make accurate readings which can easily help you to make the appropriate changes to your diet. Despite all this expertise and action, there are external factors that will surely impact your body's acid production. These external elements will substantially point out exactly how you will actually put the alkalizing meals and supplements into practice. The largest of the external elements we are talking about will be stress.

Stress is everywhere, almost global and it impacts all of us. This global problem has a very terrible effect on our body. The body works too hard to combat stress and this in turn produces even more stress! This is a vicious cycle and is propagated by a further increase in acid production. As said recently, acid is harmful to our body. An over acidic body does not run well. From the cellular perspective, the body cannot maintain the immune system. This adversely influences the circulation and the heart must compensate by working harder. As the heart beats at a faster rate to transport this sticky blood in the circulatory system, a lot of these sticky cell clumps get detached from the path and attach themselves to the walls of the arteries. This leads to a further retardation in the circulation. However, your body naturally needs blood to operate, so if the blood reaching your body cells and organs are of poor quality this can easily bring serious repercussions. Stress is acid-producing and is a killer.

There are other methods apart from diet which can easily help you in your journey to balanced pH levels. Getting adequate rest is the best method to get stress relief while at the same time taking meditation which are 2-3 times more invigorating and comfortable than real rest. Greatly reducing caffeine consumption and other similar stimulants even helps to lower body stress by eliminating these narcotics from the picture. While stress reduction is very important, increasing the consumption of meals that are alkaline in nature will reduce the effects of the acid waste in your body. Exercising is absolutely the most efficient way to get direct stress relief, and will surely help you reduce the fat stores of your body where variety of acid wastes live.

Getting more Alkaline into your diet

Diets focusing on pH balance are a unique means of examining how you eat. The requirement of the diet is keeping the ph balance of your food consumption at a level of 80 % alkalinity and 20 % acidity. The aim of this diet is to match the bloodstream ph level which is alkaline in nature. This activity can be discouraging for many people because of the fact that those foods which are high in acidity levels are the ones that they love to eat. The aim of introducing even more alkaline into your diet is to determine substantial sources of alkaline. Making a comprehensive list of foods which generate alkali will definitely help you to maximize a diet which focuses on pH balance.

Alkalizing foods give your body vitality. By their action of reducing the effects of the acidity level in your bloodstream, alkaline foods provide a "breath of fresh air" to the system which regenerates and repairs damaged cells. Diets containing high acidic foods stimulate the body, telling it to break down prematurely. The circulatory system transports these "acid bombs" through the entire system creating havoc in their wake. By finding out exactly what foods have an alkalizing effect on our body, we can introduce them into our diet in greater quantities, bringing the pH levels in our bloodstream to the optimum level. The average pH level of the human blood is anywhere between 7.3 and 7.4, levels 7 and above being considered alkaline.

Fruits and Veggies and are the most beneficial means of introducing more alkaline into your diet.

Examples of alkalizing vegetables are: kohlrabi, sea veggies, onions, rutabaga, wild greens, kale, nightshade veggies, collard greens, cauliflower, mustard greens, green beans, watercress, , carrot, garlic, mushrooms, sweet potatoes, cucumber, beet greens, celery, dandelions, green peas, pumpkin, broccoli, radishes, eggplant, lettuce, peppers, tomatoes, spinach, barley grass, beets, sprouts, chard greens, parsnips, wheat grass, alfalfa and peas.

Examples of fruits having an alkalizing effect are: raspberries, coconut, berries, currants, peaches, lemons, cantaloupe, grapes, rhubarb, avocados, cherries, strawberries, watermelon, oranges, pineapple, apples, figs, raisins, pears, honeydew, tomatoes, grapefruit, nectarines, tropical fruits, blackberries, tangerines, bananas, apricots, muskmelons, limes and dates.

Protein is possibly a challenge when you try to add even more alkaline into your diet. All animal-derived protein is acidic. It is however practicable to introduce into your diet protein that will produce alkalizing effect in your circulatory system. Some examples of alkaline proteins are: tofu, millet, tempeh, whey protein powder and chestnuts.

Food is incomplete without the sugars, spices and natural herbs which give it extra bit of character. You can add the following alkalizing condiments to your cooking efforts so as to balance your pH levels. Examples of them are: sea salt, stevia, tamari, cinnamon, mustard, curry, miso, chili pepper, ginger and all herbs.

Minerals are a necessity for ideal wellness. Observation of minerals having alkalizing consequences can make you to easily and correctly balance your blood pH. Examples of minerals having an alkalizing result on the body are: calcium, cesium, magnesium, sodium, and potassium.

There are other things which can make the addition of alkaline to your diet easier. These include: soured dairy items, mineral water, probiotic societies, lecithin granules, fresh fruit juice, molasses, veggie juices, alkaline antioxidant water, pollen, green juices and apple cider vinegar.

Your understanding of supplements and foods which add alkaline to your pH levels is only the beginning. How to execute them is your next line of action which requires dedication and planning. After you have added all these healing foods to your diet, the next thing which is easy for you to do is to test your body's pH levels by using a saliva strip examination available at most shops dealing in health foods. Restricting your pH level to any value between 7 and 8 is your target for good wellness.

Always remember that the purpose of the pH miracle diet is to ensure that your alkaline intake is higher than your acidic intake. This doesn't imply that you cannot delight the foods that are greater in acidity level. Rather, the contrary is true. Balancing of your diet must be done toward alkaline-forming foods. Keeping a correct pH balance will easily ensure that your body is operating at its ideal level.

Cooking tips for your pH balanced diet

Adopting a diet focusing on pH balance implies changing the way in which you consume and cook your food. A lot of people make this change having little or no trouble, yet for some others a diet focusing on pH balance makes takes them to the strange world of sources of fresh veggies and vegetarian protein.

You can find countless supply of alkalizing recipes for diets focusing on pH balance online and in books. You will never run out of dinner ideas if you try to find brand-new recipes every week. Although you may initially be unfamiliar with the dinners and techniques, with some practice you will certainly get used to them.

A lot of people who start begin a diet focusing on pH balance don't know where they should begin. Their diets generally contain packaged meals, meats and some other selections which form acids. Although it is fine to eat these foods from time to time, certain types of recipes and dinner options are now completely a history.

Although this may be frustrating initially, the truth is that you only need to find 10 recipes that you like and you can make easily. That's really what everybody and most of the family members use. If you attempt only 2 or 3 dinner recipes, you will truly get discouraged in the program quickly. Try a few new recipes every week to build your "portfolio" of alkalizing dinners and continue until you've got 10 meals that everyone in your household loves to consume.

Go through the list of recipes that you and all other members of your family like. Then look for even more recipes having those tastes and textures. Your family members will find it a lot easier and delicious to adjust to if you begin with foods they already like instead of suddenly introducing dandelion root, tofu and kale.

Alkalizing broth is one of the first recipes I suggest you try. There are many alternatives but in general the broth is made from distilled water and alkalizing veggies. The broth has a lot of minerals you need and can assist you in the restoration of pH balance to your body. It helps in the internal cleansing of all body organs and tissues. You can use broth as a basis for preparing even more complicated soups or use it as the first course prior to any meal.

Many fans of a diets focusing on pH balance rely on juices to help them get rid of excess acidity from their bodies. There are lots of juice recipes which are popular and can be added to your new way of eating. You can eat the juices as a fast breakfast or sometimes as a treat for the whole day. You can make many of them in a blender, so a special juicer is not really required.

Those who have children at home could be worried about finding recipes the children will certainly love. There are many vegetarian cookbooks for kids that can be adapted for the alkaline diet by substituting particular veggies. On the alkaline list are delicious fruits, such as strawberries, apples and raspberries.

There are other very alkalizing meals like sweet potatoes which become a favorite of many children once they try them and are also great for the winter season. During summer time, celery and extra fresh veggies are a great snack and you can dip them in homemade hummus or make a dip from lemon juice and mayo.

You only need a little practice and research to make alkalizing dinners that you and your family members will definitely get used to.

Green Drinks for your pH balanced diet

You probably by now have become very conscious of the importance of maintaining a diet which focuses on pH balance. As you continue to look out for more means of increasing the quantity of alkaline in your body, you've probably stumbled across the expression "green beverages". What is a green drink and how is it useful to people following a diet which focuses on pH balance?

A green drink is a simple, easy product that an individual can use to get more nutrition and alkalinity into his or her diet. The most important thing to remember with wellness and excessive weight issues is the problem caused by excessive acid in your diet. That acid collects and triggers complications in the performance of body cells. With time, the quantity of the acidity in your body raises and creates an unfavorable environment for your cells, tissues and organs. The solution is to consume alkalizing diets that have a soothing effect on your system. This will surely bring your body pH to balance and give room for your cells to work as they were ideally supposed to.

You can fill your body with alkaline foods if you consume green beverages 1 to 3 times daily. A green drink is made from sprouted grains, grasses, and some other green veggies. These will definitely provide assistance to your body and make it more alkaline. Green drinks contain natural vitamins, amino acids and minerals your body needs to correct itself.

There are various green beverages sold on the market. There are even powder types and you just mix a few spoonfuls with water daily. You can easily buy them at local health foods shops or online. However there are so many brand names to choose from, therefore you may find it difficult to narrow your choices down. The most important factor to consider in choosing a green drink is the presence of the alkaline veggie's active ingredients. Ensure that you read the component's label thoroughly. Though all of them are different, most consist of a few typical ingredients.

Kamut grass can bring down your level of cholesterol, help you burn fat and add protein to your diet. Broccoli is a strong anti-cancer food which helps you to boost your immune system and enhance your food digestion. Dandelion greens help in fat burning and lowering of cholesterol levels. In addition, they are a ready excellent source of calcium and iron. Kale contains Magnesium, Potassium, Calcium, vitamins A, C and Iron. Alfalfa sprouts helps to redistribute your body weight after your weight reduction. Green beverages contain just a few of the powerful active ingredients. Some green beverages list dozens of ingredients.

Another question you should ask yourself when you find your green beverage is, "are the active ingredients naturally grown?" Make sure that it does not contain any algae, mushroom or probiotics because all these are acidifying components. Finally, check the label very carefully for any non-nutrient item and fillers. Here is an example of a leading green beverage product.

It's the producer who determines the directions for taking green beverages. Most green beverages are taken along with water up to 4 times daily. Some are made available in the form of pills and must be taken with a lot of water. When you start taking green beverages, I advise that you take half a dosage for 7 days to familiarize your body with the effects.

Green beverages help you quickly alkalize your body by neutralizing the excess acids found in your system. A lot of people say they feel their energy instantly rising and their cravings for sugar and caffeine reduced. If you are the type who finds it difficult to perform without taking early morning coffee, try green drinks for only one week and experience the difference. Green beverages also provide support for your immune system and can easily help you minimize the amount of yeasts and contaminants in your body.

The outcomes of a diet focusing on pH balance can be felt instantly when you make take green beverages. Study the many brands that are available and then choose a brand name that looks great to you and fits the alkalizing criteria. Green beverages are a fast means of alkalizing your body and improving your wellness.

Water Ionizers and your pH balanced diet

Diets focusing on pH balance are special at bringing balance to your body. By consuming foods and beverages that are primarily alkaline, you remove the negative effects of acidic meals. People who have started the diet report that they experience fat burning, improvements in their arthritis condition, removal of concentration issues, more energy and other numerous advantages. The heart of this type of diet is alkaline foods. However, drinking of alkaline water is also essential.

Alkaline or ionized water provides your body with the correct pH it needs to make your cells to work. The pH of human body and all its cells is between 7.3 - 7.4 which is slightly alkaline. Consumption of alkaline water helps to support this system. You can produce ionized alkaline water in your own house by using a water ionizer. The water ionizer will take the water from your kitchen tap and pass it through a state-of-the-art filter which eliminates pesticides, chlorine and other contaminants. The water will then be run through an ionization chamber. In the chamber, the pre-filtered water is treated by positive and negative electrodes to break it into acid and alkaline water.

Alkaline water has a better taste and antioxidant property. It improves your body's ability to detoxify itself and deliver more oxygen to your cells. The minerals in the water are micro-clustered for better hydration. Drinking alkaline water each day will definitely assist your body to be more balanced. If you use green drinks to support your pH balanced diet, you can certainly get more efficiency by mixing them with ionized water. Using ionized water in your cooking will also produce much better tasting foods. Alkaline water will help veggies retain their natural colors when you are steaming them.

Ionized water helps to clear your body of accumulated acid and also assists in flushing contaminants out of all the body tissues and into the kidneys, where it is then ejected through the urine. If you've actually been taking a highly acidic diet and transition to a diet which focuses on pH balance we advise that you take 4 liters of ionized water daily to put your system back in order. 4 liters of ionized water every day might look like a lot, but it will be of great benefit to your health if you flush out the toxins quickly.

There are 2 water chambers in a water ionizer, one having positive electrodes and the other having negative electrodes. The negative electrodes attract the positive minerals (all of which are alkaline) and the positive electrodes attract negatively charged (acid) minerals. The alkaline minerals are calcium, potassium, magnesium and manganese. The acid minerals are chlorine, sulfur, fluoride, copper and silicon.

There's a special membrane with tiny holes between the two chambers. The holes are so small that the water molecules do not interact, but the ionized minerals can pass through the openings.
After the end of the procedure, you're going to have about 70 percent alkaline water and 30 percent acid water. The alkaline water comes through the spigot, and the acid water is expelled directly into the drain.

Water ionizers have been in use for 6 decades. They were first produced in Japan's agricultural universities. The wellness perks of ionized water were properly studied before water ionizers was made available to the Japanese public. They are now readily available to citizens in many other countries as well.

Shopping tips for your pH balanced diet

If you've decided to change to a diet focusing on pH balance, there are a few jobs ahead for you to do. Depending on exactly how much commitment you show towards the program, you could start by removing all extremely acidic foods from your cupboard and your refrigerator. If you're living with others who will not be on the diet with you, you may wish to simply take out irresistible high acid treats that you find. Whichever way, whether what you do is a "kitchen purge" or a simple removal of a few products from your shelves, you must go shopping for food.

You can shop for the pH balanced foods at any sort of supermarket. However on certain occasions, people find it a lot simpler to buy specialty items at natural food chains or health foods shops such as Whole Foods and Trader Joe's. However, if you're living in a location where you have no access to these kinds of stores, you can still conveniently collect the products you need at a popular supermarket.

Before you embark on your shopping trip, you should prepare a shopping list. You should not want to walk into the grocery store with no recollection of what you have to buy and then attempting to remember them. If you go to shop with an organized food list and the recipes opting for those dinner choices, you will buy what you need at once. A lot of the foods you are likely purchase are fresh vegetables. You should ensure that you actually need them before buying them so that your money will not be wasted on something you are not going to eat.

Always remember, when you are first starting, you don't have to make your diet 100 % alkaline. The fact is that even if you are on a strict model of diets focusing on pH balance, it is advised you maintain a balance between acid and alkaline. So when you have identified the recipes you want to try and you've prepared your grocery list, keep that fact in your mind. Examples of foods which are slightly and moderately acidic are eggs, bananas, nuts, whole grain pasta, milk, dried beans and wheat bread. There are many others and it is easy to consult a wide variety of resources on the levels of acidity found in foods. Try hard to have a balance in your everyday diet of 30 percent acid to 70 percent alkaline.

When you get to the grocery store with lists in hand, you'll see that you will probably remain along the outside of the grocery store. Usually, there are fresher meals along the walls and are more natural than the foods within the aisles. Come to think of it, all of the foods in the shop center are the processed and packaged ones. The external edges tend to display the dairy part, produce part, and the deli and meat counter.

On your shopping trip, you're going to focus on produce, veggies in particular. If you can, buy organic fruit and vegetables. However, the important thing here is that you buy the veggies and use them when you do your cooking. It is much better to use conventionally grown or frozen produce than not to use them at all.

The only strong warning is that you should avoid canned fruits and veggies. Canning procedure has great negative effects on the alkaline state of these meals. A lot of sodium is added to canned fruits and veggies. If you cannot buy fresh fruits and veggies, try to look for frozen. Many stores that don't sell organic fresh produce will definitely have organic frozen produce.

The best thing to do is to reach a balance of alkaline and acid foods as you become familiar with this style of eating. If you go for cold turkey on your favorite meals believing that you should be very strict so as to be healthy, you will revert back to your former acidic ways of eating. Try hard to begin mostly with alkaline and then easily climb further up the alkaline ladder and remove more acidic meals.

Common Mistakes people make with a pH balanced diet

By now, you certainly must have understood that it is through lowering of our dependency on foods which generate acids and increasing our consumption of alkaline generating foods that we can reach our optimal wellness. The pH scale goes from 1 to 14, where 1 means "really acidic" and 14 means "incredibly alkaline". The blood in our bloodstream possesses a tendency to go slightly alkaline at 7.35. In fact, all the foods we consume, including beverages, will eventually breakdown into alkali or acid. The body will certainly store excess quantity of acid and eliminate excess quantity of alkaline. An excessive acid quantity stored in our body will surely cluster the blood in our bloodstream, leading to fatigue and body injury on the cellular level. Too much of this type of shutdown occurring in our body will lower the immune system thereby enabling illness and ailments to set in. Retaining the balance of the pH level at 7.3-7.4 in our body will easily guarantee us sound health.

Consumption of more alkaline foods and restriction of extremely acidic foods to a reasonable level can cause preservation of a balance. By finding out which foods are alkalizing and which are acidifying, we will have the ability to make informed options. Recognizing our position on the pH scale will certainly identify exactly what changes are needed in our day-to-day routine. To track this balance we can make use of pH saliva exam strips regularly.
For those beginning a diet that focuses on pH, the initial results can be surprising.

Eating diets that do not rely on pH balance and then transitioning to one that does can sometimes be discouraging. When this happens, some dieters will try to overcompensate and begin making mistakes with this diet.

Taking excessive alkaline into their system is a common error that a lot of extremely passionate dieters will make. The role of a diet which focuses on pH balance is the provision of a long-lasting means of living. It focuses on the idea of balance. Several dieters like to address their imbalance by taking a quick fix approach which submerges them into a completely alkali intake. This is going too far with drinks and supplements which are guaranteed to increase their alkaline degrees to risky levels. As previously explained, if too much acid in the circulatory system is undesirable, so is an overabundance of alkali. Many people believe the claim that cancer cannot easily survive in an alkaline environment. True as this may be, there is absolutely nothing in our body which can easily survive for a very long time in a completely alkali environment. It is absolutely true that too many alkalis can kill us.

The key to a healthy life is a small amount of everything and a pH balanced diet is by no means an exception. Acids and alkalis are supposed to work together. Acids nurture your body and play a key role in the breaking down of materials absorbed. Your stomach is a storage tank for acids, transforming your food into energy, while alkaline is waiting in the intestinal tract to neutralize this recently stimulated product which is still to a level hot with acid.

The food materials then become metabolized, absorbed and finally passed into the bloodstream. By synchronizing these two forces, you will ensure that your body's pH degrees stay within the ideal array.

Many people who start out fail to take sufficient time to attempt to find complete listings of the pH degrees of the foods they take. Many lists can be accessed online and in various books which provide food lists that split the groups down into acids and alkalis. Selecting an extensive listing will definitely guarantee nourishment. The most preferable is a list which includes spices, herbs, supplements and condiments. Look for the fullest listing feasible which consist of those neutral foods. Taking account of how numerous acid and alkali foods are being consumed is a perfect means to guarantee proper balanced diet.

Conclusion

Thank you once again for reading The pH Balance book. By now, you should have a good understanding of how important pH balance is for a person's daily living. In this book, you have been provided with a tremendous amount of information. Reading this information was the easy part. It is now up to you to take this information and turn it into actual action and activity! Please use this information and begin improving your life and the life of others today!

CPSIA information can be obtained at www.ICGtesting.com
Printed in the USA
LVOW10s1019240416

485087LV00022B/1023/P